My Mother Has Bi Polar

Jennifer Marie Bismack

This book is dedicated to my son Dylan, my family, and to the families, educators, and healthcare professionals I hope this book helps.

Introduction

This book is for you if you have a family member or friend who was diagnosed with bi polar and want help explaining bi polar disorder to a child.

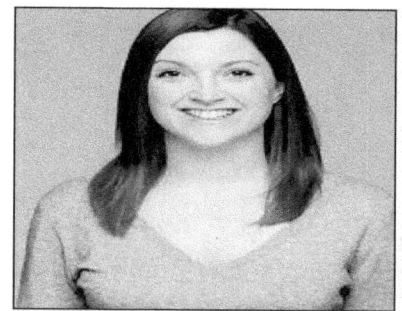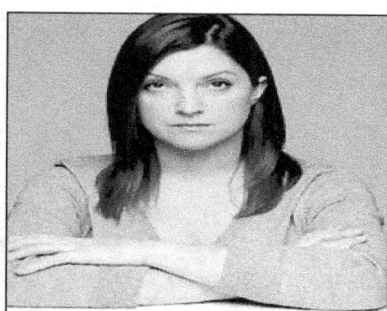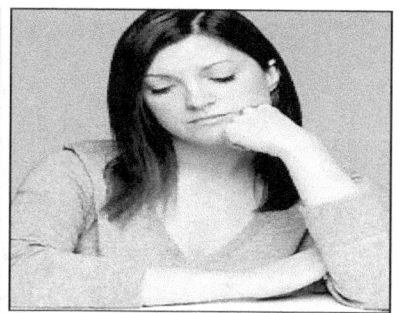

One day my mother started acting different. Her moods would be extremely happy or she would be extremely sad.

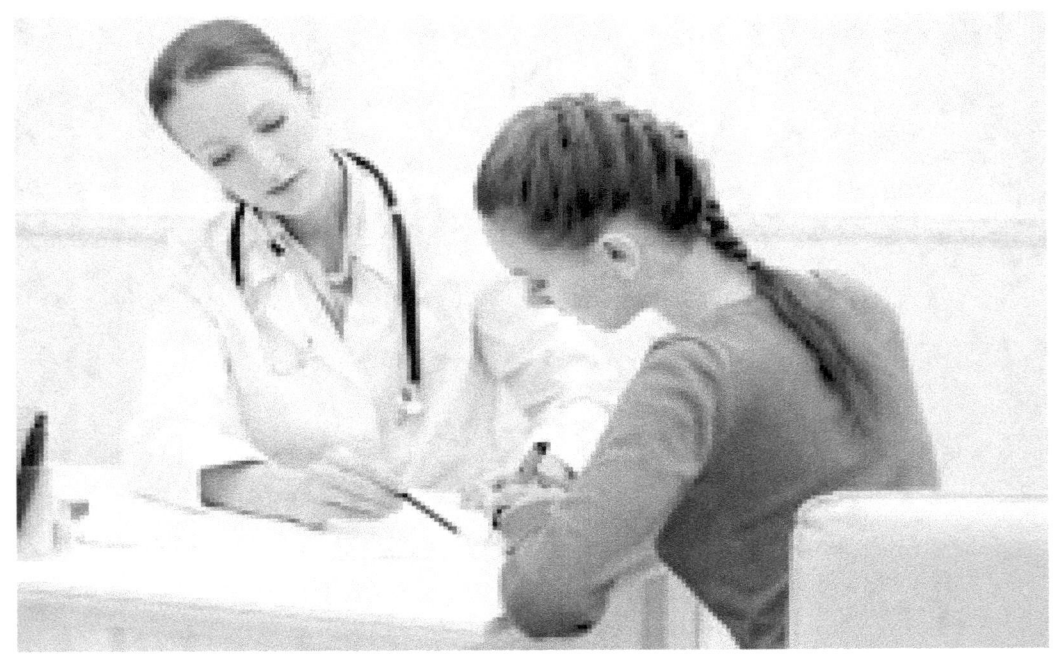

She tells me that a doctor recently diagnosed her with bi polar
and she is beginning medication to control her moods.

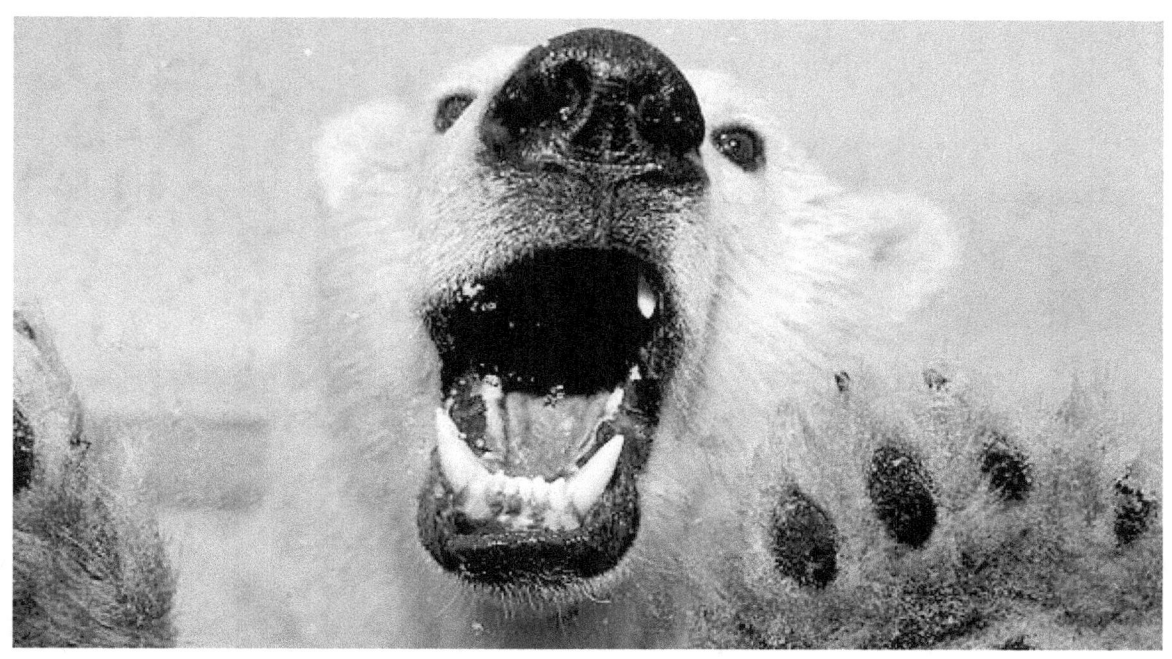

I asked my mother what exactly is bi polar? Does it mean
sometimes she acts like a mean polar bear?

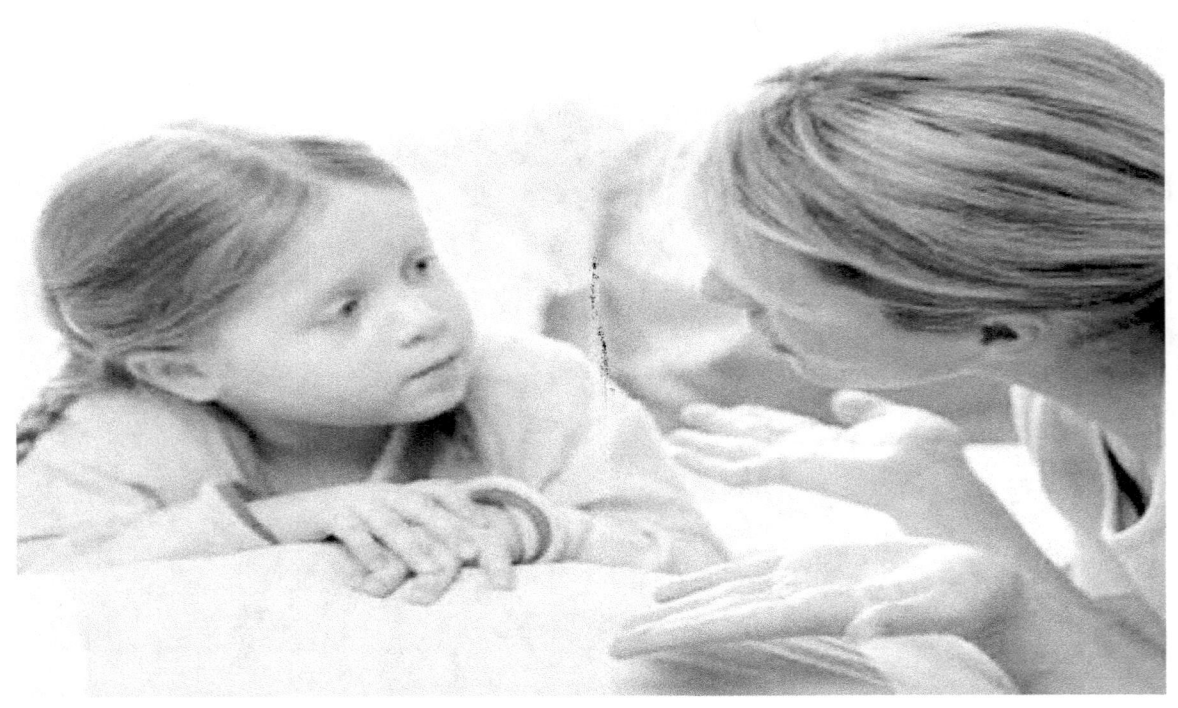

My mother told me that bi polar is also known as manic-depressive illness. It causes unusual shifts in mood, energy, activity levels, and ability to carry out day-to-day tasks.

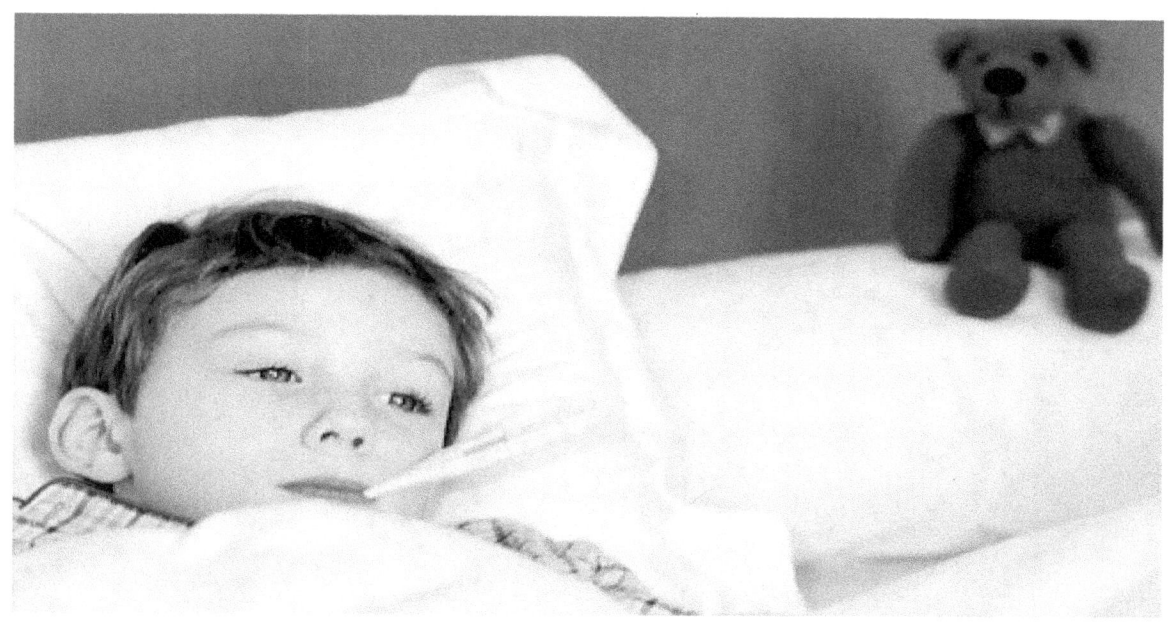

"Mom can I catch bi polar from you?" My mother said, "It's not like a cold or fever you can't just catch it in the air".

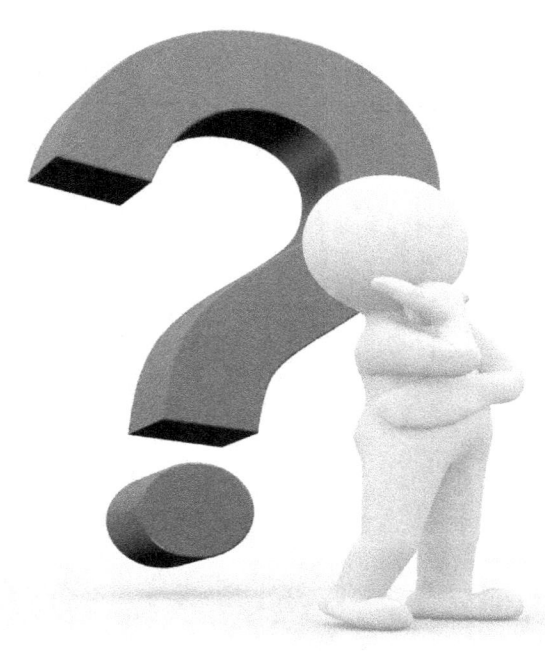

Mom then, how did you become bi polar? Mother told me there are several factors that could be the cause.

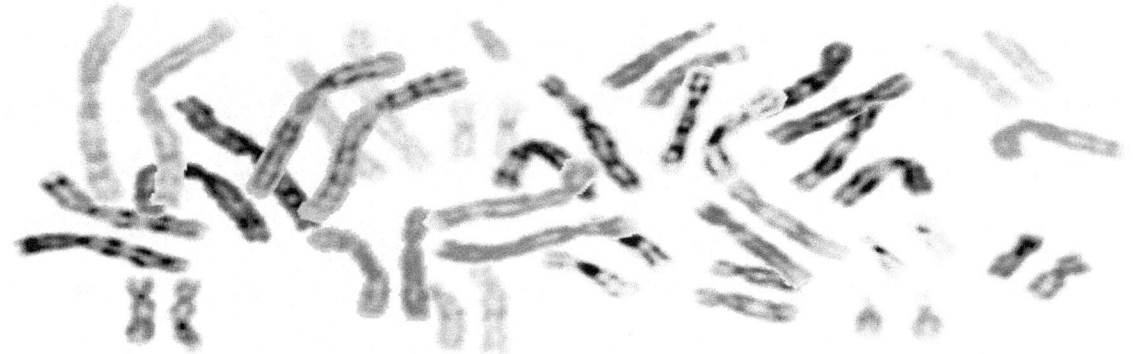

Bi polar could be caused from genes. Meaning, someone else in the family probably has bi polar. Also, abnormal brain structure and brain function could be the cause.

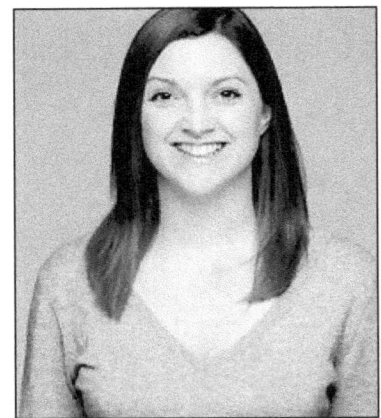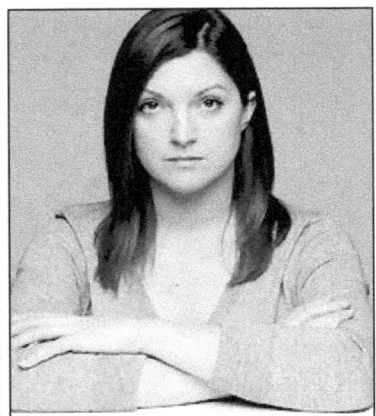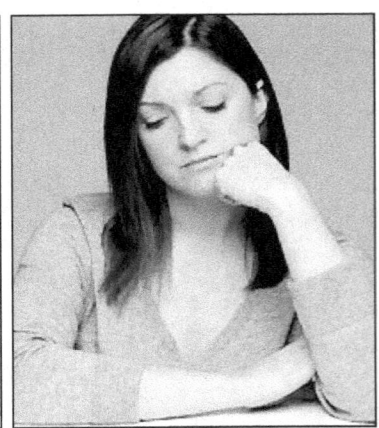

It's also, important to recognize the signs and symptoms of bi polar to understand if medication is working or not.

Symptom Domains of Bipolar Disorder

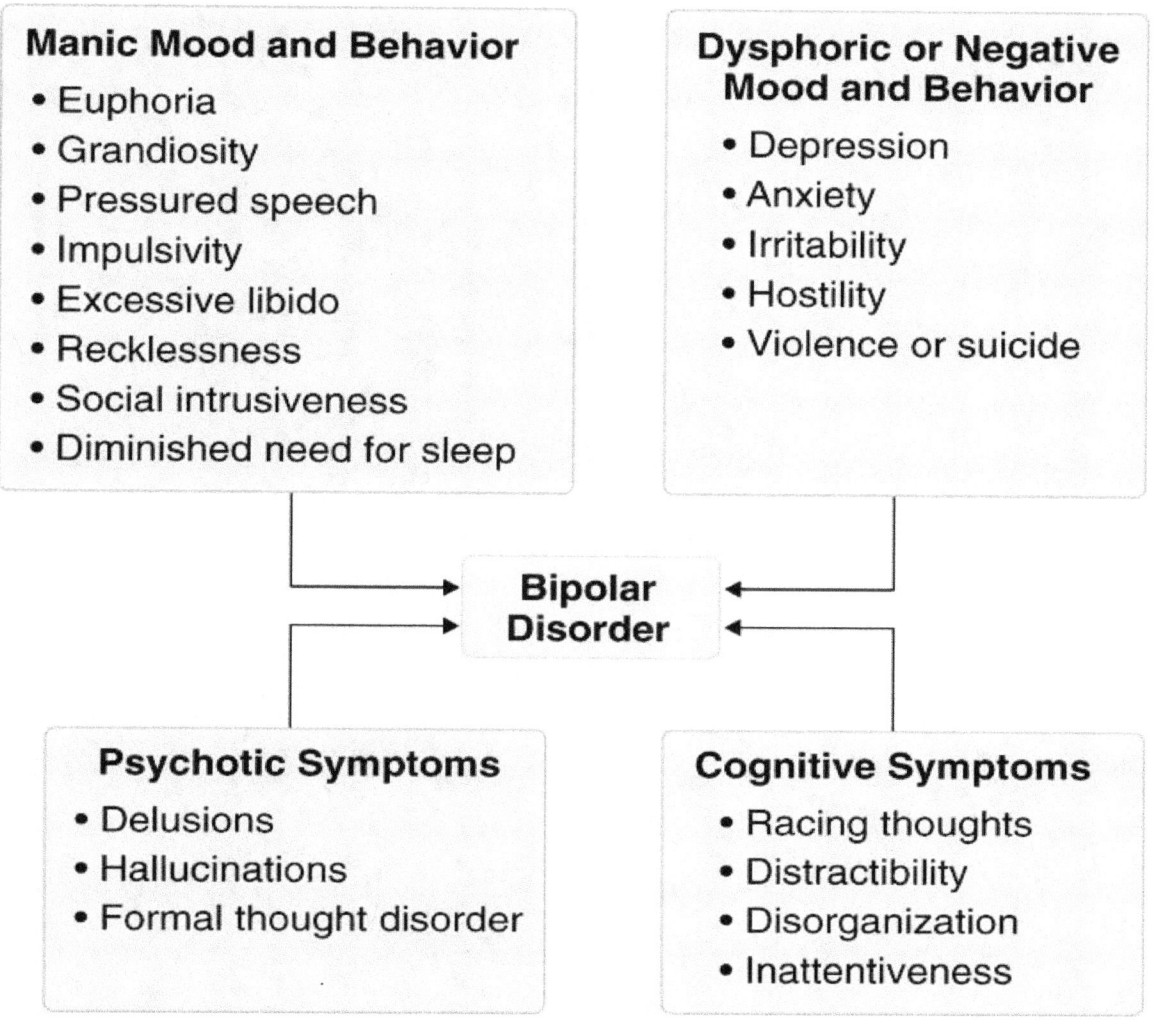

Manic Mood and Behavior
- Euphoria
- Grandiosity
- Pressured speech
- Impulsivity
- Excessive libido
- Recklessness
- Social intrusiveness
- Diminished need for sleep

Dysphoric or Negative Mood and Behavior
- Depression
- Anxiety
- Irritability
- Hostility
- Violence or suicide

Bipolar Disorder

Psychotic Symptoms
- Delusions
- Hallucinations
- Formal thought disorder

Cognitive Symptoms
- Racing thoughts
- Distractibility
- Disorganization
- Inattentiveness

What do you do if a loved one is showing behaviors or symptoms of bi polar?
You can tell your loved one your concerned about them because they are showing signs and symptoms of bi polar.

Draw a picture of you and your loved one .

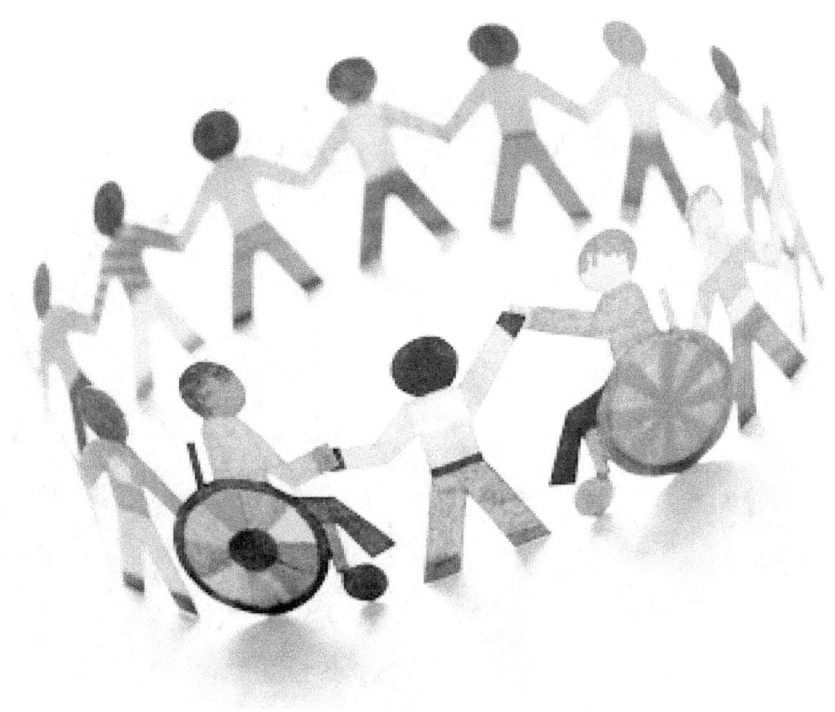

Another way to help people with a mental disability like bi polar is to include them in your life by treating them as if they don't have a disorder at all. After all they are still people.

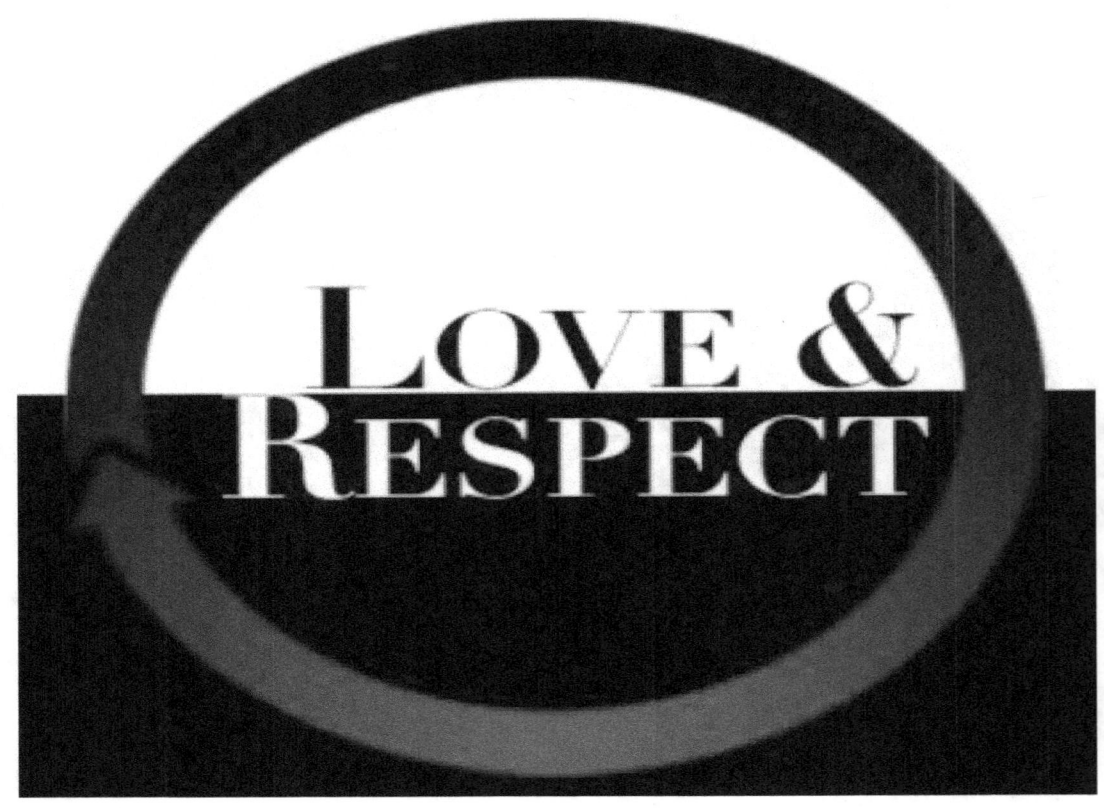

My mom says no one is perfect and everyone deserves respect, love, and to feel included. My mom went on to tell me that just because you have a disorder it does not mean that you can't do great things.

Famous People with Disabilities

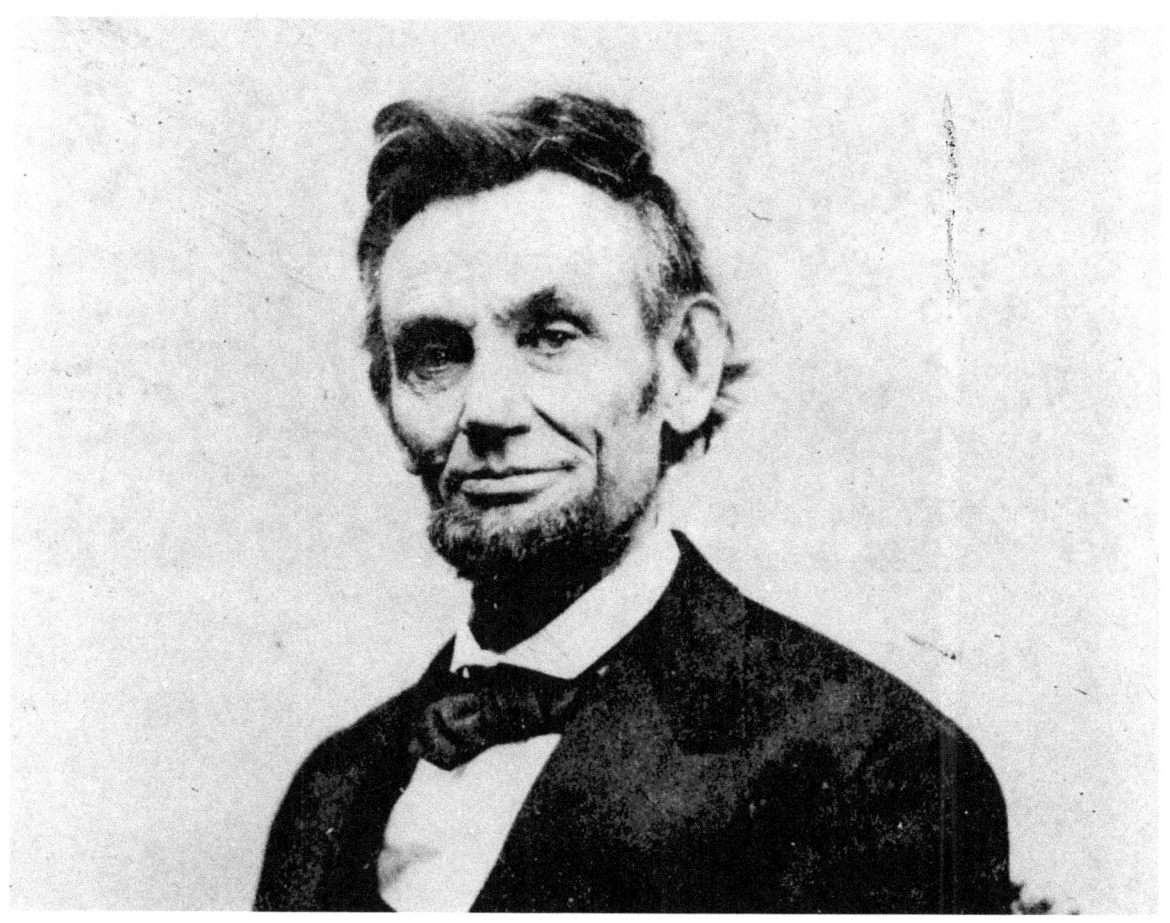

Abraham Lincoln (former President of the USA) suffered from
bi polar disorder.

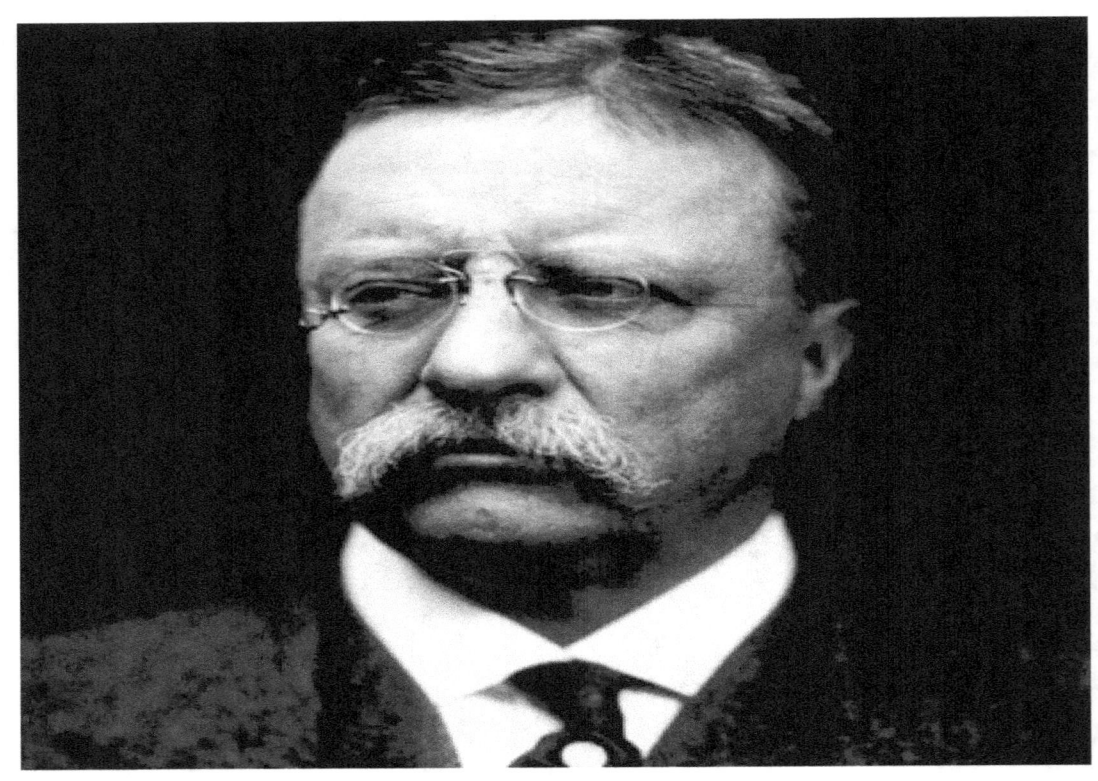

Theodore Roosevelt (former President of the USA) suffered
from bi polar disorder.

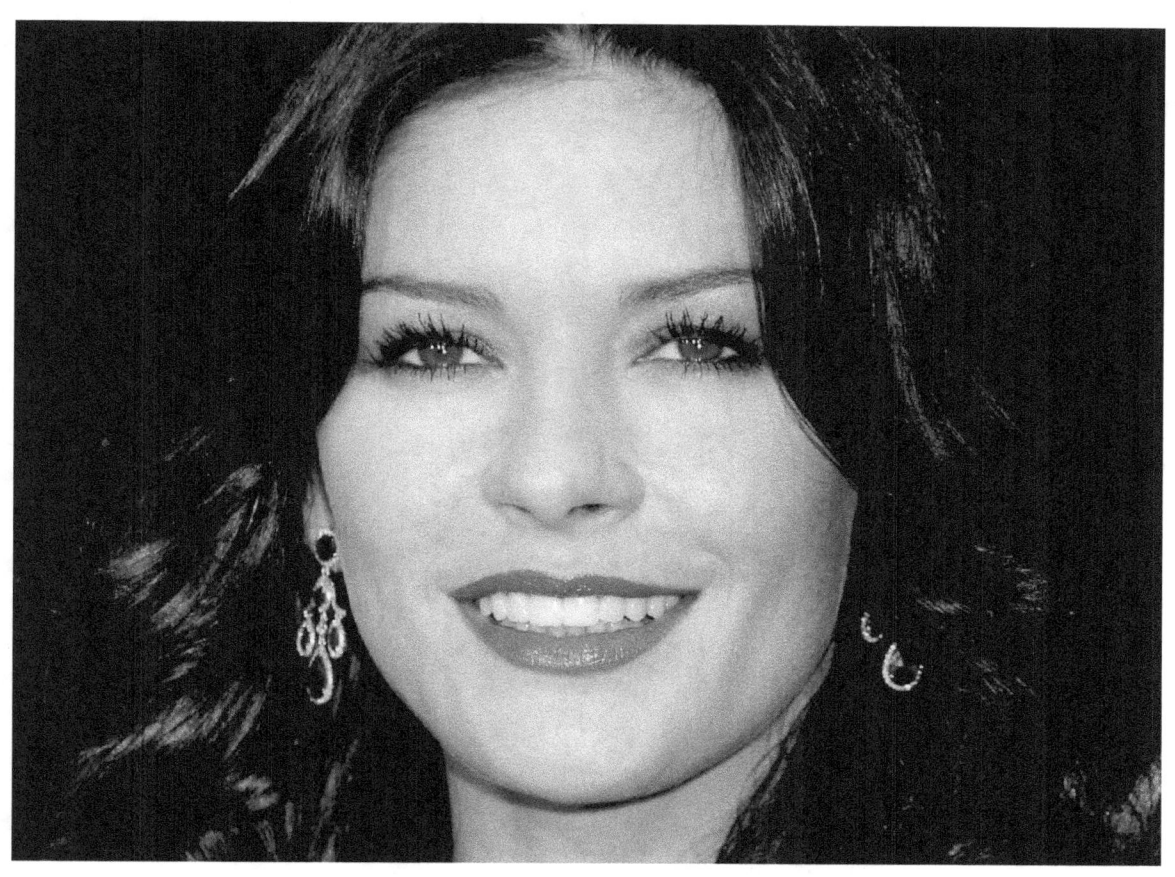

Catherine Zeta-Jones (actress) suffered from bi polar disorder.

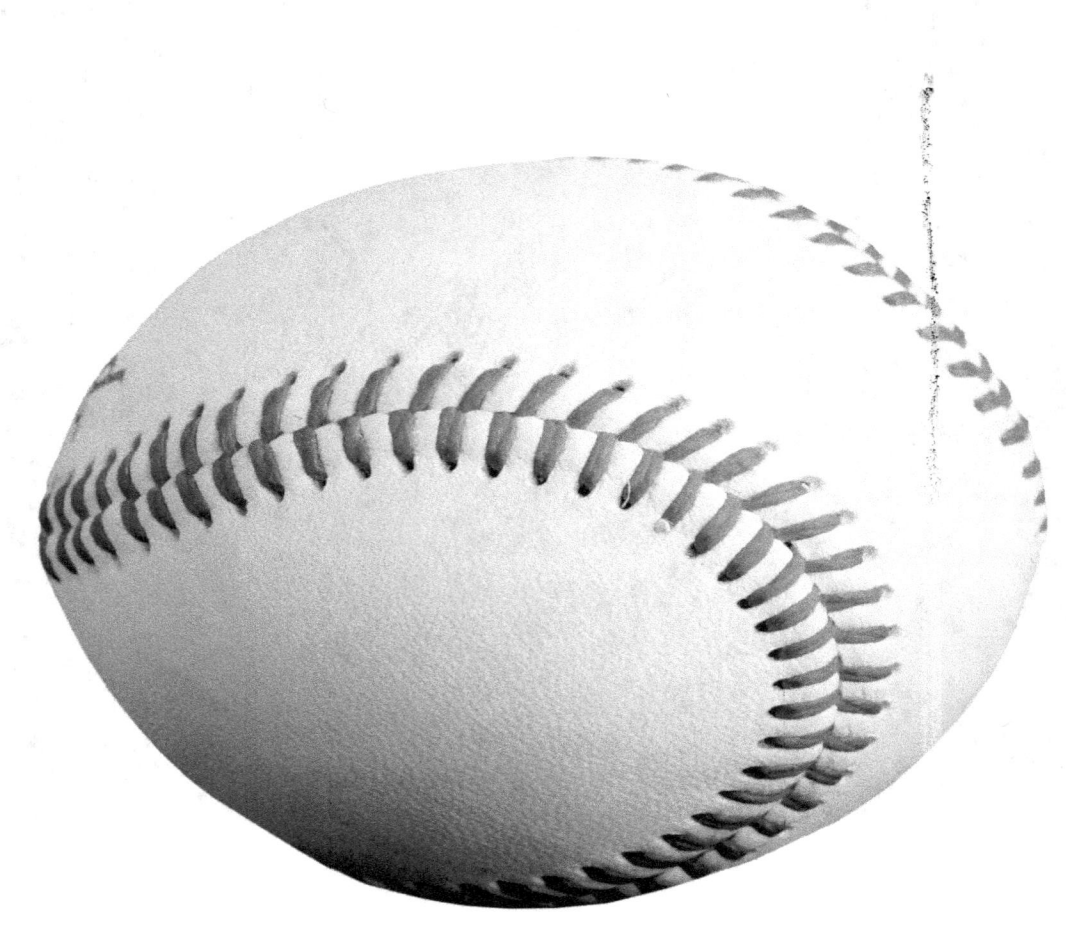

Jim Piersall (former baseball player to the Cleveland Indians) &
Darryl Strawberry (former baseball player to the New York
Yankees and New York Mets) suffered from bi polar disorder.

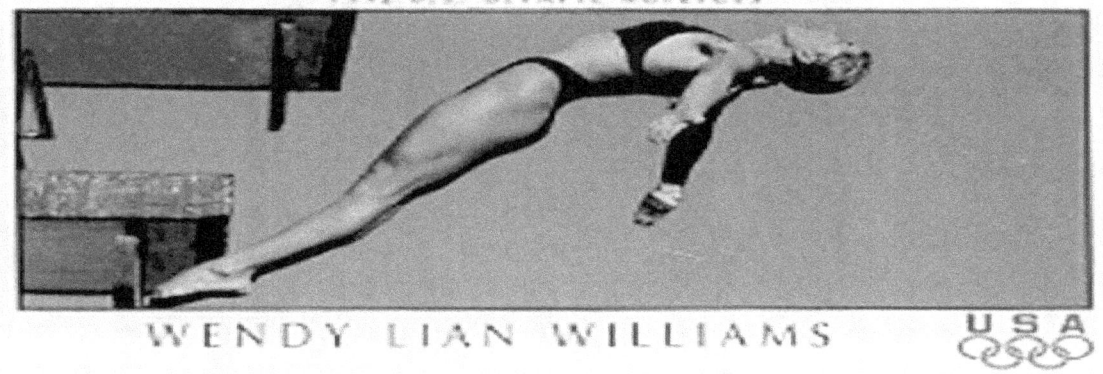

Wendy Williams (Olympic Diver) suffered from major
depression.

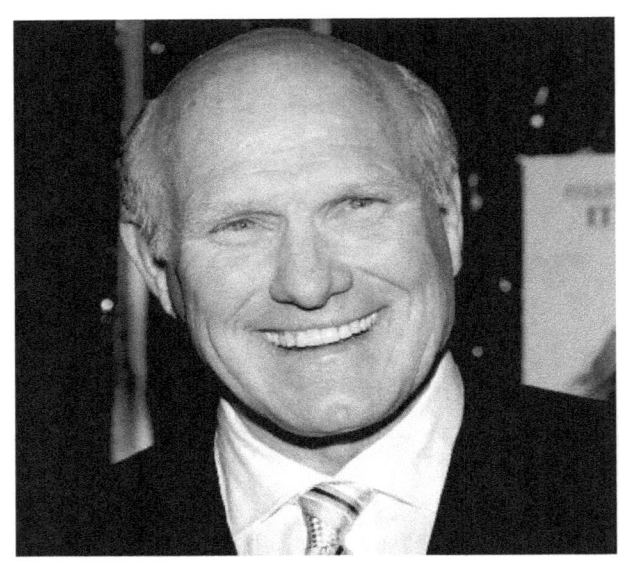

Terry Bradshaw (sports commentator & former quarterback of the Pittsburg Steelers) lived with anxiety and depression.

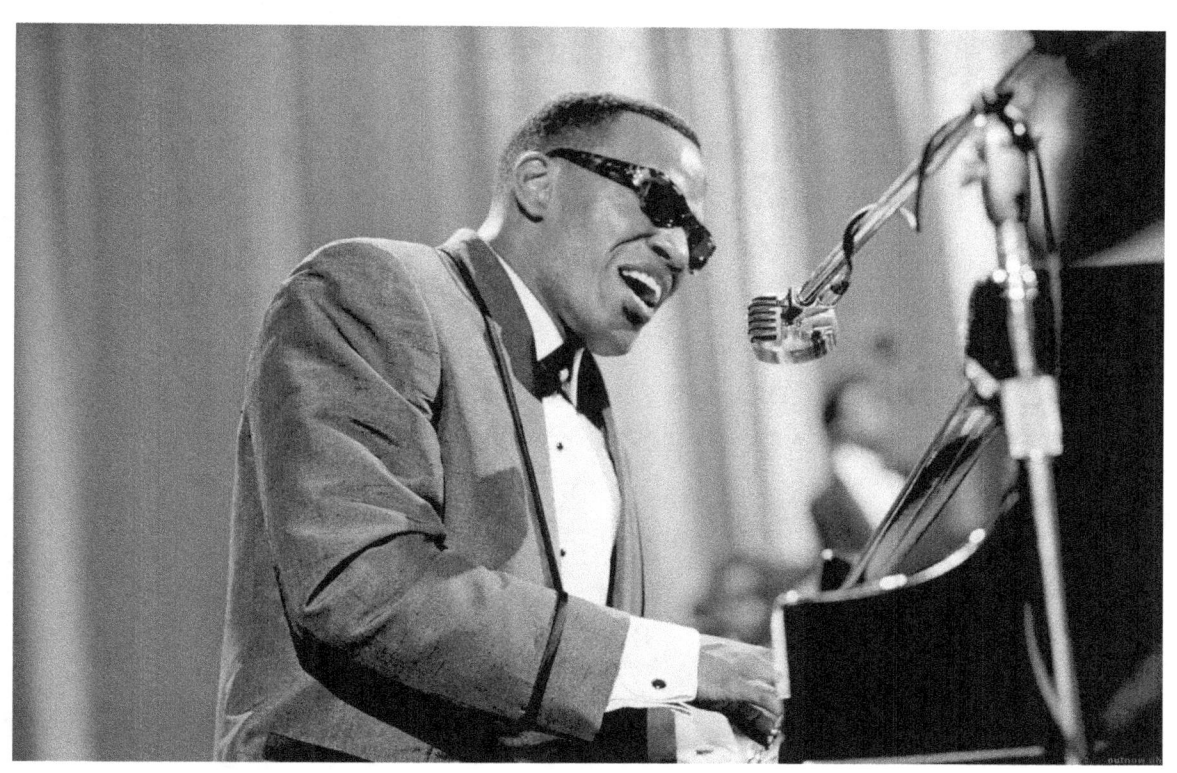

Ray Charles (singer, actor, pianist) was blind.

RECAP:

Medication can help stabilize bi polar disorder.

Bi polar causes unusual shifts in mood, energy, activity levels, and ability to carry out day-to-day tasks.

You can't catch bi polar in the air like a cold.

Bi polar disorder can be genetic or from an abnormal brain structure.

If you are around someone with bi polar disorder it is important to know the symptoms of bi polar disorder.

Treat all people with love, respect, and inclusion.

Understand that people with a disability such as bi polar disorder can go on to do great things.